Anti-Inflammatory Meat Cookbook 2021

Reset Inflammation With Meat Recipes

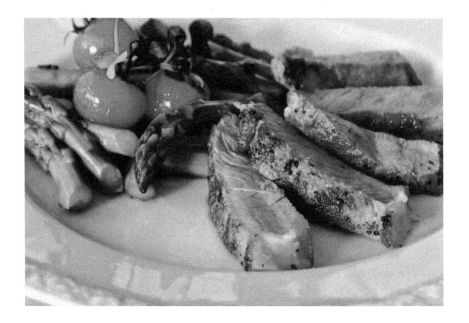

Table of Contents

Beef Meatballs in Tomato Gravy 7

Honey Glazed Beef 11

Pan Grilled Flank Steak 15

Grilled Skirt Steak 19

Spicy Lamb Curry 22

Lamb with Prunes.. 26

Lamb with Zucchini & Couscous... 29

Baked Lamb with Spinach... 32

Ground Lamb with Harissa 36

Ground Lamb with Peas 39

Roasted Leg of Lamb 43

Broiled Lamb Shoulder 46

Pan-Seared Lamb Chops... 49

Roasted Lamb Chops with Relish.. 52

Grilled Lamb Chops... 56

Lamb Burgers with Avocado Dip 59

Lamb & Pineapple Kebabs.. 63

Baked Meatballs & Scallions.. 66

Pork with Bell Pepper 70

Pork with Pineapple... 73

Spiced Pork 76

Pork Chili... 80

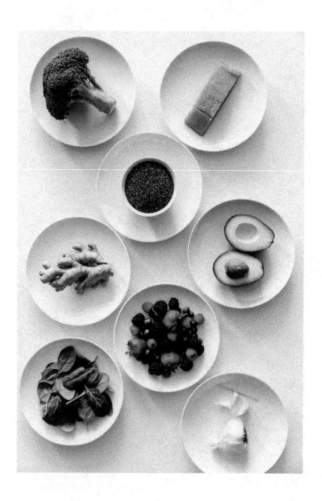

Beef Meatballs in Tomato Gravy

One with the best recipe to get ready meatballs for any lavish diner.

This recipe will be an incredible addition in the menu set of your

dinnertime meals.

Yield: 4 servings

Preparation Time: 20 minutes

Cooking Time: 37 minutes

Ingredients:

For Meatballs:1-pound lean ground beef

1 organic egg, beaten

1 tablespoon fresh ginger, minced

1 garlic oil, minced

2 tablespoons fresh cilantro, chopped finely

2 tablespoons tomato paste

1/3 cup almond meal

1 tablespoon ground cumin

Pinch of ground cinnamon

Salt and freshly ground black pepper, to taste

¼ cup coconut oilFor Tomato Gravy:2 tablespoons coconut oil

½ of small onion, chopped

2 garlic cloves, chopped

1 teaspoon fresh lemon zest, grated finely

2 cups tomatoes, chopped finely

Pinch of ground cinnamon

1 teaspoon red pepper flakes,

crushed ¾ cup chicken broth

Salt and freshly ground black pepper, to taste

¼ cup fresh parsley, choppedDirections:

1. For meatballs in a sizable bowl, add all ingredients except

oil and mix till well combined.

2. Make about 1-inch sized balls from mixture.

3. In a substantial skillet, melt coconut oil on medium heat.

4. Add meatballs and cook for approximately 3-5

minutes or till golden brown all sides.

5. Transfer the meatballs in to a bowl.

6. For gravy in a big pan, melt coconut oil on medium heat.

7. Add onion and garlic and sauté approximately 4 minutes.

8. Add lemon zest and sauté approximately 1 minute.

9. Add tomatoes, cinnamon, red pepper flakes and broth and simmer approximately 7 minutes.

10. Stir in salt, black pepper and meatballs and reduce the warmth to medium-low.

11. Simmer for approximately twenty minutes.

12. Serve hot with all the garnishing of parsley.

Nutritional Information per Serving:

Calories: 404, Fat: 11g, Carbohydrates: 27g, Fiber: 4g, Protein: 38g

Honey Glazed Beef

The best recipe for your time if you need a relatively quick meal for

family or guests. Honey glaze compliments beef very nicely.

Yield: 2-3 servings

Preparation Time: 15 minutes

Cooking Time: 12 minutes

Ingredients:2 tablespoons arrowroot flour Salt

and freshly ground black pepper, to taste

1-pound flank steak, cut into ¼-inch thick slices

½ cup plus 1 tablespoon coconut oil,

divided 2 minced garlic cloves

1 teaspoon ground ginger

Pinch of red pepper flakes,

crushed 1/3 cup organic honey

½ cup beef broth

½ cup coconut aminos

3 scallions, choppedDirections:

1. In a bowl, mix together arrowroot flour, salt and black pepper.

2. Coat beef slices in arrowroot flour mixture evenly after which get rid of excess mixture.

3. Keep aside for about 10-15 minutes.

4. For sauce in a pan, melt 1 tablespoon of coconut oil on medium heat.

5. Add garlic, ginger powder and red pepper flakes and sauté for about 1 minute.

6. Add honey, broth and coconut aminos and stir to mix well.

7. Increase the heat to high and cook, stirring continuously for around 3 minutes.

8. Remove from heat and keep aside.

9. In a large skillet, melt remaining coconut oil on medium heat.

10. Add beef and stir fry approximately 2-3 minutes.

11. Transfer the beef onto a paper towel lined plate to drain.

12. Remove the oil from skillet and return the beef into skillet.

13. Stir fry for around 1 minute.

14. Stir in honey sauce and cook approximately 3 minutes.

15. Stir in scallion and cook approximately 1 minute more.

16. Serve hot.

Nutritional Information per Serving:

Calories: 399, Fat: 15g, Carbohydrates: 28g, Fiber: 7g, Protein: 38g

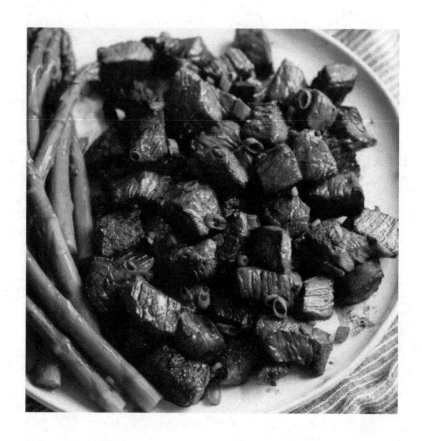

Pan Grilled Flank Steak

A pan grilled steak recipe that taste absolutely divine. This dishdoesn't require a lot of time for preparation or cooking. This is really a

delicious, simple recipe that does not have to have a long prep or cook

time. It may be the perfect meal from a long workday.

Yield: 3-4 servings

Preparation Time: 10 minutes

Cooking Time: 12-16 minutes

Ingredients:8 medium garlic cloves, crushed

1 (5-inch) piece fresh ginger, sliced thinly

1 tablespoon organic honey

¼ cup organic olive oil

Salt and freshly ground black pepper, to taste

1½ pound flank steak, trimmedDirections:

1. In a large sealable bag, mix together all ingredients except

steak.

2. Add steak and coat with marinade generously.

3. Seal the bag and refrigerate to marinate for approximately one day.

4. Remove from refrigerator and in room temperature approximately 15 minutes.

5. Lightly, grease a grill pan as well as heat to medium-high heat.

6. Discard the surplus marinade from steak and place in grill pan.

7. Cook for about 6-8 minutes from each party.

8. Remove from grill pan and keep side for around 10 min before slicing.

9. With a clear, crisp knife cut into desired slices and serve. Nutritional Information per Serving:

Calories: 432, Fat: 16g, Carbohydrates: 26g, Fiber: 5g, Protein: 35g

Grilled Skirt Steak

Coconut milk, ginger and lime marinade gives this juicy skirt steak

really a delish flavor. Definitely you would love to get this to recipe

over and over.

Yield: 4 servings

Preparation Time: 15 minutes

Cooking Time: 8-9 minutes

Ingredients:2 teaspoons fresh ginger herb, grated

finely 2 teaspoons fresh lime zest, grated finely

¼ cup coconut sugar

2 teaspoons fish sauce

2 tablespoons fresh lime

juice ½ cup coconut milk

1-pound beef skirt steak, trimmed and cut into 4-inch

slices lengthwise

Salt, to tasteDirections:

1. In a sizable sealable bag, mix together all

ingredients except steak and salt.

2. Add steak and coat with marinade generously.

3. Seal the bag and refrigerate to marinate for about 4-

12 hours.

4. Preheat the grill to high heat. Grease the grill grate.

5. Remove steak from refrigerator and discard

the marinade.

6. With a paper towel, dry the steak and sprinkle with

salt evenly.

7. Cook the steak for approximately 3½ minutes.

8. Flip the medial side and cook for around 2½-5 minutes
or

till desired doneness.

9. Remove from grill pan and keep side for approximately

5 minutes before slicing.

10. With a clear, crisp knife cut into desired slices
and serve.

Nutritional Information per Serving:

Calories: 465, Fat: 10g, Carbohydrates: 22g, Fiber: 0g, Protein: 37g

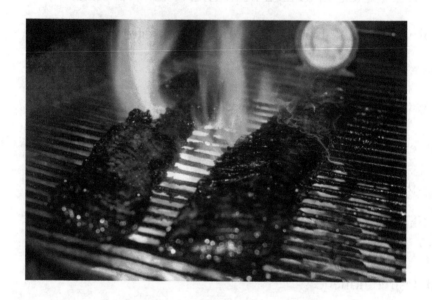

Spicy Lamb Curry

A flavorful lamb curry which is really an incredible hit for your

special occasions. This slow cooked lamb curry will surprise you

featuring its flavorful spicy flavor.

Yield: 6-8 servings Preparation

Time: 15 minutes Cooking Time:

2 hours 15 minutes Ingredients:

For Spice Mixture:4 teaspoons ground coriander

4 teaspoons ground coriander 4 teaspoons

ground cumin

¾ teaspoon ground ginger

2 teaspoons ground cinnamon

½ teaspoon ground cloves

½ teaspoon ground cardamom

2 tablespoons sweet paprika

½ tablespoon cayenne pepper

2 teaspoons chili powder

2 teaspoons saltFor Curry:1 tablespoon coconut oil

2 pounds boneless lamb, trimmed and cubed into 1-inch size

Salt and freshly ground black pepper, to

taste 2 cups onions, chopped 1¼ cups water

1 cup coconut milkDirections:

1. For spice mixture in a bowl, mix together all spices. Keep

aside.

2. Season the lamb with salt and black pepper.

3. In a large Dutch oven, heat oil on medium-high heat.

4. Add lamb and stir fry for around 5 minutes.

5. Add onion and cook approximately 4-5 minutes.

6. Stir in spice mixture and cook approximately 1 minute.

7. Add water and coconut milk and provide to some boil on

high heat.

8. Reduce the heat to low and simmer, covered for approximately 1-120 minutes or till desired doneness of lamb.

9. Uncover and simmer for approximately 3-4 minutes.

10. Serve hot.

Nutritional Information per Serving:

Calories: 466, Fat: 10g, Carbohydrates: 23g, Fiber: 9g, Protein: 36g

Lamb with Prunes

Combo of lamb and prunes is really a wonderful meal for supper.

Prunes create a perfect sweet and savory flavor in hearty lamb.

Yield: 4-6 servings

Preparation Time: fifteen minutes

Cooking Time: a couple of hours 40 minutes

Ingredients:3 tablespoons coconut oil 2

onions, chopped finely

1 (1-inch) piece fresh ginger, minced

3 garlic cloves, minced

½ teaspoon ground turmeric

2 ½ pound lamb shoulder, trimmed and cubed into 3-inch size

Salt and freshly ground black pepper, to taste

½ teaspoon saffron threads, crumbled

1 cinnamon stick

3 cups water

1 cup runes, pitted and halvedDirections:

1. In a big pan, melt coconut oil on medium heat.

2. Add onions, ginger, garlic cloves and turmeric and sauté for about 3-5 minutes.

3. Sprinkle the lamb with salt and black pepper evenly.

4. In the pan, add lamb and saffron threads and cook for approximately 4-5 minutes.

5. Add cinnamon stick and water and produce to some boil on high heat.

6. Reduce the temperature to low and simmer, covered for around 1½-120 minutes or till desired doneness of lamb.

7. Stir in prunes and simmer for approximately 20-a half hour.

8. Remove cinnamon stick and serve hot.

Nutritional Information per Serving:

Calories: 393, Fat: 12g, Carbohydrates: 10g, Fiber: 4g, Protein: 36g

Lamb with Zucchini & Couscous

One of fabulously delicious and healthy dish for whole family. This

dish is chock filled with nutrient packed

ingredients. Yield: 2 servings

Preparation Time: 15 minutes

Cooking Time: 8 minutes

Ingredients:¾ cup couscous

¾ cup boiling water

¼ cup fresh cilantro, chopped

1 tbsp olive oil

5-ounces lamb leg steak, cubed into ¾-inch

size 1 medium zucchini, sliced thinly

1 medium red onion, cut into wedges

1 teaspoon ground cumin

1 teaspoon ground coriander

¼ teaspoon red pepper flakes, crushed

Salt, to taste

¼ cup plain Greek yogurt

1 garlic herb, mincedDirections:

1. In a bowl, add couscous and boiling water and stir to combine,

2. Cover whilst aside approximately 5 minutes.

3. Add cilantro and with a fork, fluff completely.

4. Meanwhile in a substantial skillet, heat oil on high heat.

5. Add lamb and stir fry for about 2-3 minutes.

6. Add zucchini and onion and stir fry for about 2 minutes.

7. Stir in spices and stir fry for about 1 minute

8. Add couscous and stir fry approximately 2 minutes.

9. In a bowl, mix together yogurt and garlic.

10. Divide lamb mixture in serving plates evenly.

11. Serve using the topping of yogurt.

Nutritional Information per Serving:

Calories: 392, Fat: 5g, Carbohydrates: 2g, Fiber: 12g, Protein: 35g

Baked Lamb with Spinach

A stunning main course meal to the holidays. This stunning meal isn't

only mouth wateringly but super healthy too.

Yield: 6 servings

Preparation Time: 15 minutes

Cooking Time: couple of hours 55 minutes

Ingredients:2 tablespoons coconut oil

2-pound lamb necks, trimmed and cut into 2-inch pieces

crosswise

Salt, to taste

2 medium onions, chopped

3 tablespoons fresh ginger, minced

4 garlic cloves, minced

2 tablespoons ground coriander

1 tablespoon ground cumin

1 teaspoon ground turmeric

¼ cup coconut milk

½ cup tomatoes, chopped

2 cups boiling water

30-ounce frozen spinach, thawed and

squeezed 1½ tablespoons garam masala

1 tablespoon fresh lemon juice

Freshly ground black pepper, to tasteDirections:

1. Preheat the oven to 300 degrees F.

2. In a substantial Dutch oven, melt coconut oil on medium high heat.

3. Add lamb necks and sprinkle with salt.

4. Stir fry approximately 4-5 minutes or till

browned completely.

5. Transfer the lamb right into a plate and lower the heat

to medium.

6. In exactly the same pan, add onion and sauté for about 10

minutes.

7. Add ginger, garlic and spices and sauté for around

1 minute.

8. Add coconut milk and tomatoes and cook approximately 3-4 minutes.

9. With an immersion blender, blend the mix till smooth.

10. Add lamb, boiling water and salt and convey to some boil.

11. Cover the pan and transfer into the oven.

12. Bake approximately 2½ hours.

13. Now, take away the pan from oven and place on medium

heat.

14. Stir in spinach and garam masala and cook for about 3-5

minutes.

15. Stir in fresh lemon juice, salt and black pepper and

take off from heat.

16. Serve hot.

Nutritional Information per Serving:

Calories: 423, Fat: 15g, Carbohydrates: 26g, Fiber: 11g, Protein: 33g

Ground Lamb with Harissa

A delicious full meal for your table at dinnertime. Ground lamb,

harissa and spices are combined very nicely on this delicious recipe.

Yield: 4 servings

Preparation Time: 15 minutes Cooking

Time: one hour 11 minutes Ingredients:1

tablespoon extra-virgin olive oil 2 red

peppers, seeded and chopped finely 1 yellow

onion, chopped finely

2 garlic cloves, chopped finely

1 teaspoon ground cumin

½ teaspoon ground turmeric

¼ teaspoon ground cinnamon

¼ teaspoon ground ginger

1½ pound lean ground lamb

Salt, to taste

1 (14½-ounce) can diced tomatoes

2 tablespoons harissa

1 cup water

Chopped fresh cilantro, for garnishingDirections:

1. In a sizable pan, heat oil on medium-high heat.

2. Add bell pepper, onion and garlic and sauté for around 5 minutes.

3. Add spices and sauté for around 1 minute.

4. Add lamb and salt and cook approximately 5 minutes, getting into pieces.

5. Stir in tomatoes, harissa and water and provide with a boil.

6. Reduce the warmth to low and simmer, covered for about 1 hour.

7. Serve hot while using garnishing of harissa. Nutritional Information per Serving:

Calories: 441, Fat: 12g, Carbohydrates: 24g, Fiber: 10g, Protein: 36g

Ground Lamb with Peas

A best tasting spiced ground lamb recipe for supper. Surely all so

want to eat this spiced dish of lamb and

veggies. Yield: 4 servings

Preparation Time: 15 minutes

Cooking Time: 55 minutes

Ingredients:1 tablespoon coconut

oil 3 dried red chilies

1 (2-inch) cinnamon stick

3 green cardamom pods

½ teaspoon cumin seeds

1 medium red onion, chopped

1 (¾-inch) piece fresh ginger, minced

4 garlic cloves, minced

1½ teaspoons ground coriander

½ teaspoon garam masala

½ teaspoon ground cumin

½ teaspoon ground turmeric

¼ teaspoon ground nutmeg

2 bay leaves

1-pound lean ground lamb

½ cup Roma tomatoes, chopped

1-1½ cups water

1 cup fresh green peas, shelled

2 tablespoons plain Greek yogurt, whipped

¼ cup fresh cilantro, chopped

Salt and freshly ground black pepper, to tasteDirections:

1. In a Dutch oven, melt coconut oil medium-high heat.

2. Add red chilies, cinnamon stick, cardamom pods and cumin seeds and sauté for around thirty seconds.

3. Add onion and sauté for about 3-4 minutes.

4. Add ginger, garlic cloves and spices and sauté for around thirty seconds.

5. Add lamb and cook approximately 5 minutes.

6. Add tomatoes and cook approximately 10 min.

7. Stir in water and green peas and cook, covered

approximately 25-thirty minutes.

8. Stir in yogurt, cilantro, salt and black pepper and cook for

around 4-5 minutes.

9. Serve hot.

Nutritional Information per Serving:

Calories: 430, Fat: 10g, Carbohydrates: 22g, Fiber: 6g, Protein: 26g

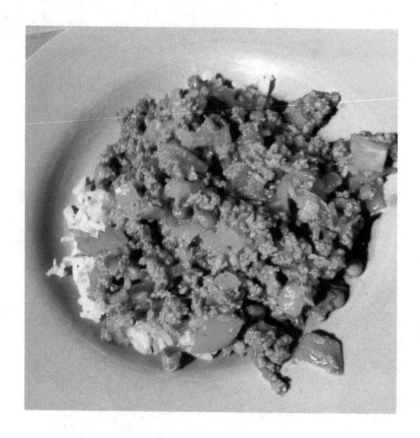

Roasted Leg of Lamb

One of best dish for weeknight dinners. Slow roasting gives leg of

lamb a great perfection of flavoring.

Yield: 8 servings

Preparation Time: 15 minutes Cooking

Time: 75-100 minutes Ingredients:1/3

cup fresh parsley, minced 4 garlic cloves,

minced

1 teaspoon fresh lemon zest, grated finely

1 tablespoon ground coriander

1 tablespoon ground cumin

1 teaspoon ground cinnamon

1 teaspoon ground turmeric

1 tablespoon sweet paprika

½ teaspoon allspice

20 saffron threads, crushed

1/3 cup essential olive oil

1 (5-pound) leg of lamb, trimmedDirections:

1. In a bowl, mix together all ingredients except lamb.

2. Coat the leg of lamb with marinade mixture generously.

3. With a plastic wrap, cover the leg of lamb and refrigerate to marinate for about 4-8 hours.

4. Remove from refrigerator and keep in room temperature for about a half-hour before roasting.

5. Preheat the oven to 350 degrees F. Arrange the rack inside the center of the oven.

6. Lightly, grease a roasting pan make a rack inside roasting pan.

7. Place the lower limb of lamb in the rack in prepared roasting pan.

8. Roast for approximately 75-100 minutes or till desired doneness, rotating once inside the middle way.

Nutritional Information per Serving:

Calories: 392, Fat: 12g, Carbohydrates: 20g, Fiber: 4g, Protein: 37g

Broiled Lamb Shoulder

A super-healthy and flavorful dish for supper table. This healthy and

delicious dish is prepared with no fuss in less time.

Yield: 10 servings

Preparation Time: 10 minutes

Cooking Time: 8-10 minutes

Ingredients:2 tablespoons fresh ginger,

minced 2 tablespoons garlic, minced

¼ cup fresh lemongrass stalk, minced

¼ cup fresh orange juice

¼ cup coconut aminos

Freshly ground black pepper, to taste 2-

pound lamb shoulder, trimmedDirections:

1. In a bowl, mix together all ingredients except lamb

shoulder.

2. In a baking dish, squeeze lamb shoulder and coat the

lamb with half in the marinade mixture generously.

3. Reserve remaining mixture.

4. Refrigerate to marinate for overnight.

5. Preheat the broiler of oven. Place a rack inside a broiler pan and arrange about 4-5-inches from heating unit.

6. Remove lamb shoulder from refrigerator and remove excess marinade.

7. Broil approximately 4-5 minutes from both sides.

8. Serve with all the reserved marinade like a sauce. Nutritional Information per Serving:

Calories: 250, Fat: 19g, Carbohydrates: 2g. Fiber: 0g, Protein: 15g

Pan-Seared Lamb Chops

A hearty lamb chops recipe using the flavorful touch of warm spices.

This recipe will probably be perfect for dinner and launch too.

Yield: 4 servings

Preparation Time: 10 minutes

Cooking Time: 4-6 minutes

Ingredients:4 garlic cloves, peeled

Salt, to taste

1 teaspoon black mustard seeds, crushed finely

2 teaspoons ground cumin

1 teaspoon ground ginger

1 teaspoon ground coriander

½ teaspoon ground cinnamon

Freshly ground black pepper, to

taste 1 tablespoon coconut oil

8 medium lamb chops, trimmedDirections:

1. Place garlic cloves onto a cutting board and sprinkle with salt.

2. With a knife, crush the garlic till a paste forms.

3. In a bowl, mix together garlic paste and spices.

4. With a clear, crisp knife, make 3-4 cuts on both side in the chops.

5. Rub the chops with garlic mixture generously.

6. In a large skillet, melt butter on medium heat.

7. Add chops and cook for approximately 2-3 minutes per side or till desired doneness.

Nutritional Information per Serving:

Calories: 443, Fat: 11g, Carbohydrates: 27g, Fiber: 4g, Protein: 40g

Roasted Lamb Chops with Relish

Entertain all your family members with these satisfying roasted lamb

chops. These delicious roasted lamb chops are infused using the taste

of spices, yogurt fresh lime.

Yield: 4 servings

Preparation Time: 15 minutes

Cooking Time: half an hour

Ingredients:

For Lamb Marinade:4 garlic cloves, chopped

1 (2-inch) piece fresh ginger, chopped

2 green chilies, seeded and chopped

1 teaspoon fresh lime zest

2 teaspoons garam masala

1 teaspoon ground coriander

1 teaspoon ground cumin

½ teaspoon ground cinnamon

1 teaspoon coconut oil, melted

2 tablespoons fresh lime juice

6-7 tablespoons plain Greek yogurt

1 (8-bone) rack of lamb, trimmed

2 onions, slicedFor Relish:½ of garlic herb, chopped

1 (1-inch) piece fresh ginger, chopped

¼ cup fresh cilantro, chopped

¼ cup fresh mint, chopped

1 green chili, seeded and chopped

1 teaspoon fresh lime zest

1 teaspoon organic honey

2 tablespoons fresh apple juice

2 tablespoons fresh lime juiceDirections:

1. For chops in a very mixer, add all ingredients except yogurt, chops and onions and pulse till smooth.

2. Transfer the mixture in a large bowl with yogurt and stir to combine well.

3. Add chops and coat with mixture generously.

4. Refrigerate to marinate for approximately 24 hours.

5. Preheat the oven to 375 degrees F. Linea roasting pan with a foil paper.

6. Place the onion wedges in the bottom of prepared roasting pan.

7. Arrange rack of lamb over onion wedges.

8. Roast approximately half an hour.

9. Meanwhile for relish in the blender, add all ingredients and pulse till smooth.

10. Serve chops and onions alongside relish.

Nutritional Information per Serving:

Calories: 439, Fat: 17g, Carbohydrates: 26g, Fiber: 10g, Protein: 41g

Grilled Lamb Chops

A really simple and easy to organize grilled lamb chops which might

be rich in flavors. This recipe is a great option for barbecue parties.

Yield: 4 servings

Preparation Time: 10 min

Cooking Time: 6 minutes

Ingredients:1 tablespoon fresh ginger, grated

4 garlic cloves, chopped roughly 1 teaspoon

ground cumin

½ teaspoon red chili powder

Salt and freshly ground black pepper, to taste

1 tbsp essential olive oil

1 tablespoon fresh lemon juice

8 lamb chops, trimmedDirections:

1. In a bowl, mix together all ingredients except chops.

2. With a hand blender, blend till a smooth mixture forms.

3. Add chops and coat with mixture generously.

4. Refrigerate to marinate for overnight.

5. Preheat the barbecue grill till hot. Grease the grill grate.

6. Grill the chops for approximately 3 minutes per side. Nutritional Information per Serving:

Calories: 227, Fat: 12g, Carbohydrates: 1g, Fiber: 0g, Protein: 30g

Lamb Burgers with Avocado Dip

A winner and delicious burger recipe for whole family. These burgers

are wonderful when with smooth and silky textured avocado dip.

Yield: 4-6 servings

Preparation Time: 20 minutes

Cooking Time: 10 minutes

Ingredients:

For Burgers:1 (2-inch) piece fresh ginger, grated

1-pound lean ground lamb 1 medium onion, grated

2 minced garlic cloves

1 bunch fresh mint leaves, chopped finely

2 teaspoons ground coriander

2 teaspoons ground cumin

½ teaspoon ground allspice

½ teaspoon ground cinnamon

Salt and freshly ground black pepper, to taste

1 tbsp essential olive oilFor Dip:3 small cucumbers, peeled and grated

1 avocado, peeled, pitted and chopped

½ of garlic oil, crushed

2 tablespoons fresh lemon juice

2 tablespoons olive oil

2 tablespoons fresh dill, chopped finely

2 tablespoons chives, chopped finely

Salt and freshly ground black pepper, to tasteDirections:

1. Preheat the broiler of oven. Lightly, grease a broiler pan.

2. For burgers in a big bowl, squeeze the juice of ginger.

3. Add remaining ingredients and mix till well combined.

4. Make equal sized burgers from your mixture.

5. Arrange the burgers in broiler pan and broil

approximately 5 minutes per side.

6. Meanwhile for dip squeeze the cucumbers juice in

a bowl.

7. In a blender, add avocado, garlic, lemon juice and oil and

pulse till smooth.

8. Transfer the avocado mixture in a bowl.

9. Add remaining ingredients and stir to mix.

10. Serve the burgers with avocado dip.

Nutritional Information per Serving:

Calories: 462, Fat: 15g, Carbohydrates: 23g, Fiber: 9g, Protein: 39g

Lamb & Pineapple Kebabs

One from the delicious recipe of lamb and pineapple kebabs using a

tasty layer of char. Fresh mint provides a refreshing touch to those

kebabs.

Yield: 4-6 servings

Preparation Time: 15 minutes

Cooking Time: 10 minutes

Ingredients:1 large pineapple, cubed into 1½-inch size, divided

1 (½-inch) piece fresh ginger, chopped

2 garlic cloves, chopped

Salt, to taste

16-24-ounce lamb shoulder steak, trimmed and cubed into

1½-inch size

Fresh mint leaves coming from a bunch

Ground cinnamon, to tasteDirections:

1. In a blender, add about 1½ servings of pineapple, ginger,

garlic and salt and pulse till smooth.

2. Transfer the amalgamation right into a large bowl.

3. Add chops and coat with mixture generously.

4. Refrigerate to marinate for about 1-2 hours.

5. Preheat the grill to medium heat. Grease the grill grate.

6. Thread lam, remaining pineapple and mint leaves onto pre-soaked wooden skewers.

7. Grill the kebabs approximately 10 min, turning occasionally.

Nutritional Information per Serving:

Calories: 482, Fat: 16g, Carbohydrates: 22g, Fiber: 5g, Protein: 377g

Baked Meatballs & Scallions

A recipe of lamb meatballs that is filled with flavor and aroma. Baked

meatballs pair nicely with all the crispy tips of braised scallions.

Yield: 4-6 servings

Preparation Time: 20 min

Cooking Time: 35 minutes

Ingredients:

For Meatballs:1 lemongrass stalk, outer skin peeled and chopped

1 (1½-inch) piece fresh ginger, sliced

3 garlic cloves, chopped

1 cup fresh cilantro leaves, chopped roughly

½ cup fresh basil leaves, chopped roughly

2 tablespoons plus 1 teaspoon fish sauce

2 tablespoons water

2 tablespoons fresh lime juice

½ pound lean ground pork

1-pound lean ground lamb

1 carrot, peeled and grated

1 organic egg, beatenFor Scallions:16 stalks scallions, trimmed

2 tablespoons coconut oil,

melted Salt, to taste

½ cup waterDirections:

1. Preheat the oven to 375 degrees F. Grease a baking dish.

2. In a blender, add lemongrass, ginger, garlic, fresh herbs, fish sauce, water and lime juice and pulse till chopped finely.

3. Transfer the amalgamation in a bowl with remaining ingredients and mix till well combined.

4. Make about 1-inch balls from mixture.

5. Arrange the balls into prepared baking dish in a single layer.

6. In another rimmed baking dish, arrange scallion stalks in a very single layer.

7. Drizzle with coconut oil and sprinkle with salt.

8. Pour water in the baking dish 1nd with a foil paper cover it tightly.

9. Bake the scallion for around a half-hour.

10. Bake the meatballs for approximately 30-35 minutes. Nutritional Information per Serving:

Calories: 432, Fat: 13g, Carbohydrates: 25g, Fiber: 8g, Protein: 40g

Pork with Bell Pepper

This stir fry not simply tastes wonderful but additionally is packed

with nutritious benefits. Fresh lime juice intensifies the taste with this

stir fry.

Yield: 4 servings

Preparation Time: 15 minutes

Cooking Time: 13 minutes

Ingredients:1 tablespoon fresh ginger, chopped finely

4 garlic cloves, chopped finely

1 cup fresh cilantro, chopped and divided

¼ cup plus 1 tbsp olive oil, divided

1-pound tender pork, trimmed, sliced thinly

2 onions, sliced thinly

1 green bell pepper, seeded and sliced thinly

1 tablespoon fresh lime juiceDirections:

1. In a substantial bowl, mix together ginger, garlic, ½ cup of

cilantro and ¼ cup of oil.

2. Add pork and coat with mixture generously.

3. Refrigerate to marinate approximately a couple of hours.

4. Heat a big skillet on medium-high heat.

5. Add pork mixture and stir fry for approximately 4-

5 minutes.

6. Transfer the pork right into a bowl.

7. In the same skillet, heat remaining oil on medium heat.

8. Add onion and sauté for approximately 3 minutes.

9. Stir in bell pepper and stir fry for about 3 minutes.

10. Stir in pork, lime juice and remaining cilantro and cook for

about 2 minutes.

11. Serve hot.

Nutritional Information per Serving:

Calories: 429, Fat: 19g, Carbohydrates: 26g, Fiber: 9g, Protein: 35g

Pork with Pineapple

A wonderfully delicious recipe which will surely impress a meat

lover. Pineapple compliments pork tenderloin in the wonderful way.

Yield: 4 servings

Preparation Time: 15 minutes

Cooking Time: 14 minutes

Ingredients:2 tablespoons coconut oil

1½ pound pork tenderloin, trimmed and cut into bite-

sized pieces

1 onion, chopped

2 minced garlic cloves

1 (1-inch) piece fresh ginger, minced

20-ounce pineapple, cut into chunks

1 large red bell pepper, seeded and

chopped ¼ cup fresh pineapple juice

¼ cup coconut aminos

Salt and freshly ground black pepper, to tasteDirections:

1. In a substantial skillet, melt coconut oil on high heat.

2. Add pork and stir fry approximately 4-5 minutes.

3. Transfer the pork right into a bowl.

4. In exactly the same skillet, heat remaining oil on medium heat.

5. Add onion, garlic and ginger and sauté for around 2 minutes.

6. Stir in pineapple and bell pepper and stir fry for around 3 minutes.

7. Stir in pork, pineapple juice and coconut aminos and cook for around 3-4 minutes.

8. Serve hot.

Nutritional Information per Serving:

Calories: 431, Fat: 10g, Carbohydrates: 22g, Fiber: 8g, Protein: 33g

Spiced Pork

One from the absolute delicious dish of spiced pork. Slow cooking

helps you to infuse the spice flavors in pork very

nicely. Yield: 6 servings

Preparation Time: fifteen minutes

Cooking Time: 1 hour 52 minutes

Ingredients:1 (2-inch) piece fresh ginger, chopped

5-10 garlic cloves, chopped 1 teaspoon ground

cumin

½ teaspoon ground turmeric

1 tablespoon hot paprika

1 tablespoon red pepper flakes

Salt, to taste

2 tablespoons cider vinegar

2-pounds pork shoulder, trimmed and cubed into 1½-inch

size

2 cups domestic hot water, divided

1 (1-inch wide) ball tamarind pulp

¼ cup olive oil

1 teaspoon black mustard seeds, crushed

4 green cardamoms

5 whole cloves

1 (3-inch) cinnamon stick

1 cup onion, chopped finely

1 large red bell pepper, seeded and choppedDirections:

1. In a food processor, add ginger, garlic, cumin, turmeric, paprika, red pepper flakes, salt and cider vinegar and pulse till smooth.

2. Transfer the amalgamation in to a large bowl.

3. Add pork and coat with mixture generously.

4. Keep aside, covered for around an hour at room temperature.

5. In a bowl, add 1 cup of warm water and tamarind and make aside till water becomes cool.

6. With the hands, crush the tamarind to extract the pulp.

7. Add remaining cup of hot water and mix till well

combined.

8. Through a fine sieve, strain the tamarind juice inside a bowl.

9. In a sizable skillet, heat oil on medium-high heat.

10. Add mustard seeds, green cardamoms, cloves and cinnamon stick and sauté for about 4 minutes.

11. Add onion and sauté for approximately 5 minutes.

12. Add pork and stir fry for approximately 6 minutes.

13. Stir in tamarind juice and convey with a boil.

14. Reduce the heat to medium-low and simmer 1½ hours.

15. Stir in bell pepper and cook for about 7 minutes.

Nutritional Information per Serving:

Calories: 435, Fat: 16g, Carbohydrates: 27g, Fiber: 3g, Protein: 39g

Pork Chili

A great bowl of healthy chili with the amazing addition of Bok choy.

This healthy chili is tasty, spicy and refreshing on the same time.

Yield: 8 servingsPreparation Time: 15 minutes

Cooking Time: 1 hour

Ingredients:2 tablespoons extra-virgin organic olive oil

2-pound ground pork

1 medium red bell pepper, seeded and chopped

1 medium onion, chopped

5 garlic cloves, chopped finely

1 (2-inch) part of hot pepper, minced

1 tablespoon ground cumin

1 teaspoon ground turmeric

3 tablespoon chili powder

½ teaspoon chipotle chili powder

Salt and freshly ground black pepper, to taste

1 cup chicken broth

1 (28-ounce) can fire-roasted crushed tomatoes

2 medium Bok choy heads, sliced

1 avocado, peeled, pitted and choppedDirections:

1. In a sizable pan, heat oil on medium heat.

2. Add pork and stir fry for about 5 minutes.

3. Add bell pepper, onion, garlic, hot pepper and spices and stir fry for approximately 5 minutes.

4. Add broth and tomatoes and convey with a boil.

5. Stir in Bok choy and cook, covered for approximately twenty minutes.

6. Uncover and cook approximately 20-half an hour.

7. Serve hot while using topping of avocado.

Nutritional Information per Serving:

Calories: 402, Fat: 9g, Carbohydrates: 18g, Fiber: 6g, Protein: 32g

CPSIA information can be obtained
at www.ICGtesting.com
Printed in the USA
LVHW010456140521
687424LV00003B/175